MASSAGE

IN A BOX

BHARTI VYAS

About the Author

Bharti Vyas grew up surrounded and influenced by ancient Eastern philosophies and traditional Asian methods of healthcare. She is an influential name in the health and beauty field, with a successful clinic in London and her own popular beauty products. A qualified acupuncturist, she has extensive knowledge of mineral therapy and aromatherapy.

MASSAGE

IN A BOX

BHARTI VYAS

with contributing editors
Claire Haggard and Jane Warren

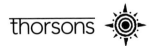

Thorsons
An Imprint of HarperCollins*Publishers*
77-85 Fulham Palace Road
Hammersmith
London W6 8JB

This edition published in 2003
10 9 8 7 6 5 4 3 2 1

Text for this edition derived from Simply Radiant,
Simply Ayurveda and Beauty Wisdom

Bharti Vyas asserts the moral right to be identified
as the author of this work

A catalogue record for this book is available from the British Library

ISBN 0-00-715366-X

Printed and bound in Hong Kong

IMPORTANT:

While largely beneficial for most health conditions, massage and acupressure should not be undertaken when a person is under the influence of alcohol or drugs, or is suffering from some medical conditions.

Never use essential oils undiluted as part of a massage or acupressure session. If you are pregnant, or have recently given birth, consult your doctor before using aromatherapy oils or embarking on a massage programme.

Massage and acupressure do not replace conventional diagnosis and treatment for any ailment or disease. If in doubt, consult a doctor.

CONTENTS

INTRODUCTION

Touch is the essence of massage. How our body feels to us is much more important than how it looks or what it does. The key to knowing how our body feels is the simple joy of giving and receiving touch. It is the medium through which we communicate on a non-verbal level. Touch has been shown to be vital for newborns of all species to thrive, and skin-to-skin contact affects our health throughout all stages of our lives.

Our hands are highly sensitive and powerful healing tools, with the ability to influence the workings of our bodies. When applying certain massage techniques using different parts of our hands, we stimulate the circulation and help the body drain away toxic fluids through the lymph system (see page 82). This eases tension, and brings a sense of balance and wellbeing.

During massage and acupressure, the body's natural energy centres, known as acupoints, are balanced and revitalized. Acupoints are key markers on a network of invisible meridians or channels, through which the body's vital energy, or chi, flows. When the flow becomes blocked, ill health follows; when it flows abundantly and freely, we enjoy good health and wellbeing. In acupuncture, the points are stimulated with needles, a practice that is carried out by a professionally qualified therapist. Acupressure is acupuncture's little sister – no needles are used, and instead the points are stimulated using the fingers. Acupressure is safe to perform yourself, but do take note of the cautions listed on page 4. In this section you will also find a diagram showing the meridians and acupoints on the body, along with instructions on locating them and the health benefits when you stimulate them.

Acupressure is rooted in Chinese medicine and is thought to be several thousand years old. In India, a similar philosophy of health developed, based on the chakra system (see page 59). The life force, or prana, runs through the body's seven principal energy vortices, or chakras. When the chakras are healthy and in sync, we are well in mind, body and spirit. One of the practical applications of this philosophy is the ancient Indian healing system known as Ayurveda. On cards 10–20 and 26–30 are massages popular in Ayurveda – plus information on discovering your type, or dosha (see page 54).

Give yourself some time to work through this book and use the cards. It may take a little time to get your touch right and locate precisely some acupressure points, but your intention to give and receive healing is what makes massage work – tuning into yourself or your partner's body using these time-honoured techniques will relax and energize you, and help keep you in good health throughout your life.

How to Use the Book and Cards

Cards 1, 2 and 3 explain simple massage and acupressure techniques to begin with – fingerballing, palming, pinching and feathering. You can use each of them to varying degrees to add some variety to your massage routines. If your skin is healthy and not oversensitive, it is better to use the more intense techniques such as pinching and fingerballing – palming and feathering are gentler strokes.

Cards 4 to 30 then take you through a body massage that you can practise on yourself or a friend or partner. You can also enjoy using aromatherapy or Ayurvedic oils to enhance the experience (see pages 54 and 56 to choose the oils that will enhance the power of your massage). You can choose a short sequence for the face or hands, or set aside an evening to treat yourself to a head-to-toe massage.

1 HOW MASSAGE WORKS

Massage is an ancient therapy that boosts the circulation and helps our bodies eliminate waste more effectively. For thousands of years, this healing art has been used to prevent ill health and soothe specific ailments. As well as being an enjoyable experience, it has its beauty benefits, too, improving muscle tone by stimulating the body's soft tissue – the muscles, ligaments and tendons.

Drench and Drain

Your life depends on your body being able to deliver regular supplies of nourishment and oxygen to every tiny cell, and remove the rubbish that would otherwise pollute your tissues. We have in our heart and blood vessels both a powerful mechanism and an extensive circuit to achieve this, backed up by a network of neighbouring lymphatic vessels.

The lymphatic system (which also maintains a fluctuation reserve of water in between the cells) acts as the skin's internal irrigation service, sluicing out potential pollutants and keeping the conditions in the tissues as salubrious as possible.

The main drainage point for the lymphatic system is located in the groin, which is one of the reasons why we treat the face and body together: it helps to clear the system as a whole. The lymphatic system works away in the shadow of the blood circulation, closer to the skin's surface. A network of tiny tubes hoovers up debris and leaked fluids from the spaces between the cells and conveys it to filtering stations, known as lymph nodes, which remove all the harmful wastes and bacteria. These eventually flow into the veins, enabling the missing fluids to be returned to the blood. In this way the lymphatic system plays a vital role in maintaining a healthy internal environment. However, since it relies on the massaging effect of the muscles and a good breathing action rather than a central pump to propel the fluid around the body, it is prone to become sluggish.

Fluid wastes are circulating around our systems all the time without necessarily doing any harm. When fluid wastes settle in our tissues, however, they can cause havoc. This is known as 'stagnation' – when the resulting toxic sediment causes progressive deterioration of the tissue unless action is taken to disturb and dispose of it. Problems also arise if the amount of water required by the body for efficient circulation is drastically reduced, as is the case with chronic constipation and crash dieting. The face is particularly vulnerable to these problems due to the patchy coverage and precise configuration of blood vessels. The good news is that we are able to boost our circulation and keep stagnation at bay with the help of massage, which encourages lymphatic flow and drainage and so corrects any imbalances – and every little helps.

Massage For Life: Benefits You See and Feel

After a few weeks of using your massage programme, which will cleanse and invigorate your lymphatic system, these internal changes will begin to reveal themselves, both as improvements in your appearance and in increased energy levels. Regular massage can:

- Transform skin tone on the body and face, and increase the capacity of dry skin to absorb nourishment
- Clear skin and reduce blocked pores, limiting the damage caused by overactive sebaceous oil glands
- Banish eye bags by flushing out lymph fluid from the under-eye area and reduce 'panda' eyes syndrome by stimulating circulation
- Maintain healthy joints by protecting the surrounding cartilage from damage caused by stagnating fluid
- Help curb facial blemishes and acne rosacea, as well as reduce the occurrence of broken capillaries on the body
- Encourage the body's largest organ, the skin, to renew itself more frequently

2 GETTING STARTED

When starting a massage session, be sure to prepare the space. If you are using oils, have a clean towel and container to hand, and cover chairs and beds with a cotton sheet. Do not drink coffee or alcohol in the time prior to the session, but keep a large glass of water by you to drink after the massage has ended – see below. You might like to try the bathing and relaxation spa recipes given below to add extra relaxation to your session. Once you have chosen the massage to perform from the cards or this book, turn to page 15 to choose the oils that will increase the healing effects of your massage – you can even mix oils to target specific body areas and ailments as well as creating personal blends that will boost your wellbeing.

Oils for Massage

Working with oils during a massage is not only more pleasurable, but also enhances the relaxing qualities of the massage. As you massage, the oils will moisturise the skin deeply, while using aromatherapy oils or Ayurvedic blends (see pages 54 and 56) will allow you to treat specific ailments, as well as boost the qualities of the massage. For example, a night-time face massage to help you sleep can be even more effective if you add lavender essential oil to your massage base oil as it is traditionally good for relaxation. To give an energy boost to a vitality massage, you could choose a light citrus oil such as neroli. When working with a partner, the right oils will add to the sensuality and togetherness of the massage experience.

How to Mix an Aromatherapy Oil

Essential oils should always be diluted in a base, or carrier, oil such as almond or grapeseed (see the list overleaf). The healing plant extracts that each contains are strong and if applied neat their properties can damage the skin. (Lavender oil and tea tree oil, however, have been used neat, without being diluted, to treat specific ailments such as a burn or athlete's foot, but not in the context of massage.) If you are allergic to nuts, stick to vegetable-based oils such as avocado or olive oil.

An aromatherapy oil for massage will constitute about 1–3 per cent of essential oil in a base oil. Mix 100ml of the base oil with 20–60 drops of the essential oil you choose in a cup. You can choose more than one essential oil to create your personal blend, but be sure never to exceed the 1–3 per cent ratio.

While aromatherapy oils should be used unheated, once you have created the blend, always rub between your palms to warm it for a few seconds before applying to the skin. To store any remaining oil, pour carefully into dark-blue or brown glass containers with a screwtop or dropper lid and store in a cool, dark place to avoid oxidation, which will reduce their effectiveness. Discard any unused oils after six months.

Choosing a Massage Oil

Just as the lymphatic system cleanses the body from the inside, you can promote its rejuvenating and purifying effect on the skin by choosing an appropriate massage oil. Try out a variety to see which you like best. Some are heavier and more sticky than others, which won't suit oilier skins. Grapeseed is often a popular choice for people with oily or normal skins due to its light consistency.

Base Oils

Almond
Sesame
Grapeseed
Coconut

Essential Oils

For Relaxation
Lemon balm
Cinnamon leaf
Geranium
Jasmine
Juniper
Lavender (true)
Mandarin
Peppermint
Orange
Rose
Sandalwood
Rosemary
Vetiver
Ylang ylang
Clary sage

Relaxation Recipe
15 drops rose oil
10 drops lavender oil
100ml sweet almond oil

For Dry Skin

Wheatgerm
Avocado
Peach or apricot kernel
Peanut oil
Jojoba
Olive oil

For Energy
Cardamom
Citronella
Grapefruit
Ginger
Lavender (spike)
Lemongrass
Nutmeg
Cumin
Pine
Neroli

Energy Recipe
15 drops grapefruit oil
5 drops citronella oil
100ml grapeseed oil

Water for Life

Water is an important part of massage. Internally, it's needed to cleanse our system and flush out toxins, which are released during a massage. Externally, water therapies can be used to complement a massage treatment.

Drinking Water

Our bodies are composed of over 80 per cent water. While we do need to drink up to two litres of water a day for optimum bodily function, drinking water after a massage is especially important. As the lymphatic system gathers up toxins during the massage, these need to be eliminated. Drinking a large glass of water after your treatment will help the liver and kidneys expel waste. Sipping the water slowly in the moments after a massage also promotes relaxation. Don't, however, drink iced water – this is too much of a shock to the system after a warm massage!

Hydrotherapy

You can practise this simple hydrotherapy treatment before you begin a massage. It involves using hot and cold water alternately to help restore skin tone and boost the cleansing effects of massage by stimulating circulation. Apply an ice-cold compress – a suitably sized towel or piece of cloth soaked through in iced water and then wrung out – to the area of your body you will be massaging. Hold it in place for 40 seconds, then blast with warm water from the shower for three minutes. Repeat up to five times.

Beauty Massage Spa

This brilliant stress-buster leaves your skin gleaming, banishes the day's stress and nourishes your body with the rich minerals of Dead Sea salt. You'll need a quiet evening – and the bathroom all to yourself. Repeat this routine once or twice a week.

If you suffer from skin problems, such as psoriasis or eczema, or have sleeping difficulties, make the spa massage a daily routine.

Stress, diet, injury and illness can all have a traumatizing effect on the body's tissues, which initially makes them less able to absorb and make use of the minerals contained in the salts. It is therefore important to take more frequent baths to begin with, until you notice some improvement.

Ingredients
Dead Sea salts
Base oil (see page 15)
An exfoliating cream or scrub (if you prefer, you can make your own using 2 tablespoons of finely ground oatmeal mixed with 1 tablespoon of almond oil)
Mineral shower gel
Lavender or sandalwood essential oils (optional)

1. Relax

Create a relaxed ambience in your bathroom. Tidy and clean up before you begin, set the scene with the soft glow of candlelight and play soothing music of your choice. Have a flannel and large towel to hand.

2. Massage your scalp

Oil and massage your scalp thoroughly – see Cards 16–20. When you've done this, wrap your hair in a towel or shower cap.

3. Exfoliate

Exfoliation boosts your circulation, loosens any dead skin cells and moisturizes your skin in preparation for the mineral therapy in Step 4.

Don't exfoliate more than once a week; if you don't need to exfoliate now, just skip this step and apply a light film of almond oil to your skin before you bathe.

Rub the exfoliant over your trunk, arms, legs, neck, face and behind your ears. Pay special attention to hard skin on elbows, knees, soles and heels. Massage into fingernails and toenails, working right into the cuticles. Shower off the exfoliator.

4. Mineral therapy

Run a warm bath. Check that the temperature of the water is pleasantly warm, so you feel inclined to linger. Water that is too hot will stimulate rather than relax you – and it can dehydrate and slacken the skin, as well as damage fragile capillaries. Add three or four handfuls of Dead Sea salts plus a squirt of mineral shower gel to the bath water. If you suffer from a dry skin condition such as eczema, start with a teaspoon of salts, increasing gradually as tolerance builds up.

Submerge yourself in the bath for at least 30 minutes. For the first 10 minutes, just soak and relax. Then remove your towel or shower cap and briefly dip your head and wet your face.

5. Body rubbing

Take your flannel and gently rub your face and then all over your body, especially on areas of hard skin. Use the cloth to push back the cuticles around your finger and toenails, and then relax until the 30 minutes is up.

To complete your spa, shower off the salts and towel yourself dry. Apply a good mineral body lotion to further hydrate your skin. Go straight to bed or relax under a warm cover. You will still have oil in your hair from the scalp massage, so protect your pillow with an old towel. As you sleep, the therapy will go on working overnight, assisting the repair process that is underway when your body is at rest.

When you wash your hair the next morning, shampoo twice with a mineral shampoo; leave the second shampoo on for 10 minutes before rinsing thoroughly.

Dry Skin Brushing

Dry skin brushing with a natural bristle brush before your bath or shower boosts skin circulation and enhances the lymph-clearing effects of massage. Aiding the flow of lymph, the brushing also allows toxins to leave the body more rapidly. Always brush in the direction of the heart and avoid broken or sore areas of skin.

Skin Secrets

As you learn to massage, and with practice, you will become more aware of the condition of your skin, and that of the person whom you are massaging. You will also become more adept at choosing the appropriate base massage oils for your skin type (see page 15). Below is a list of common skin imperfections, with suggested treatments should you wish or need to take action.

Liver Spots

Liver spots are caused by cumulative ultraviolet radiation. They appear on the most exposed parts of the body, such as the face and hands, in later years as a result of pigmentation changes beneath the skin.

What can be done

- As soon as you notice pigmentation marks developing, start wearing a high-protection sunscreen at all times. Apply a sun block if you are going to be exposed to intense sunlight.

- A vitamin B-complex supplement, supported by a balanced diet, may help.
- Hormonally related pigmentation should correct itself, but if the patches do not disappear within six months, see your doctor to check hormone levels. If the problem persists, you can opt for professional treatment to stimulate circulation to the basal layer of the skin, which can help to disperse the pigment.

Vitiligo

This is the absence of pigment in small, defined areas of skin. It can be caused by shock or stress, which produces a chemical that interferes with the function of melanin cells. The illness has also an occasional side effect of bleaching dark skins.

What can be done
- Total sun block is essential to protect affected areas.
- Cosmetic camouflage can be very effective.

Skin Tags

These are small, greyish growths that usually appear on the neck and eyelids, and sometimes on the back and midriff. These often accompany hormonal changes in middle age.

What can be done
- They can be treated painlessly and successfully with high-current electrolysis.

Moles

These small, raised clusters of pigmented cells beneath the skin develop during adolescence and are mostly inconspicuous and trouble-free, although facial moles with protruding hairs can cause problems if the follicle becomes irritated and inflamed.

What can be done
- Laser treatment is an effective method of removing moles, which does not leave a scar.
- Always consult your doctor before having moles removed or if unusual-looking moles appear, or if a long-standing mole starts to change its shape or increase in size.

Warts

Warts are caused by an infectious virus, which invades the skin via tiny cracks and fissures resulting in abnormal growth of skin cells. They occur on the hands, knees, feet (the inward-growing verrucas) and on the face.

What can be done

- If you don't want to wait for them to disappear of their own accord, treat them homoeopathically or buy a suitable preparation at a chemist.

Healing Recipes for the Skin

Stabilizing Face Mask

Good for:
- Sensitive skin
- Premature wrinkles
- Acne rosacea

Ingredients
1 heaped teaspoon gram flour
1 teaspoon double cream
2 teaspoons water
A pinch of salt

Gram, or chickpea, flour, a cosmetic staple in Indian households, is prized for its ability to nourish and cleanse the skin. Buy it at health shops, larger supermarkets and Asian stores.

Double cream has a composition not unlike a rich moisturizer, and is naturally well endowed with vitamin A, as well as useful amounts of vitamins D and E – a natural skin food.

Mix the ingredients together to make a thick cream. Apply to the skin, leave for 10 minutes and rinse off.

Healing Mask

Good for:
• Spots and mild acne

Ingredients
2 teaspoons honey
1 teaspoon fine sea salt
1 teaspoon turmeric

Honey dislodges dead skin cells and is valued for its soothing, healing, emollient and mild antiseptic properties. Use the runny variety. However, if you are allergic to pollen and grasses, avoid masks with honey as an ingredient.

Salt is a powerful cleanser and neutralizer of bacteria, as well as a natural exfoliator. Turmeric is renowned for its healing powers in India, where it is sprinkled onto cuts to speed up the clotting and repair process. Combined with other ingredients in a mask, it is very effective in clearing the complexion.

Mix together to make a thick paste. Apply to spots every evening and leave on for up to 30 minutes, or overnight. When the spots have cleared, this treatment can be used preventatively as a face pack once a month.

Eczema Mask

Ingredients
2 teaspoons gram flour
2 teaspoons almond oil
1 teaspoon salt

Mix together to form a smooth lotion. Apply to affected areas, and leave for 10 minutes.

3 MASSAGE TECHNIQUES

Acupressure Massage

Acupressure is the application of deep fingertip or thumb pressure at specific points on the body. This ancient Oriental system of treatment is easy to learn and takes only a short time to perform. It can be used to promote general good health and wellbeing, as well as to relieve a wide range of common ailments.

Many masseurs use acupressure as a part of massaging. The effect of acupressure is to fine-tune our internal machinery, increase energy levels and resistance to illness, while enhancing, directly or indirectly, different aspects of our appearance. It is easy to see the connection between a sluggish digestive system or inefficient circulation and the health of the skin, or how a constant level of pain or stiffness could distort your posture as well as your facial expression. You can help to relieve such problems by administering your own acupressure treatment.

According to Chinese medicine, our energy flows along established channels, or meridians. These are connected to the organs and systems of the body. When this flow of energy, or chi, is interrupted, it creates an imbalance within the body, which is manifested on the outside as a problem or symptom. By stimulating the pressure points of the meridians, which lie just beneath the surface of the skin (acupressure points or acupoints), the natural harmony can be restored.

Meridians

THE BODY'S MERIDIANS, OR
ENERGY PATHS THAT CHANNEL
OUR VITAL ENERGY, OR CHI.

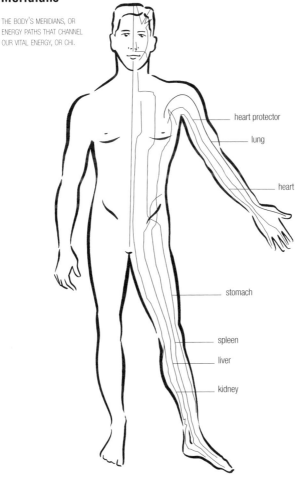

heart protector

lung

heart

stomach

spleen

liver

kidney

Applying Pressure

It can take time to locate acupressure points exactly. With practice, you will be able to hone in on the spot instantly – although at first you may feel at sea and wonder what it is you are supposed to be feeling for. A mild pain sensation will often confirm that you are in the right place. A small amount of pain is actually curative, and any discomfort will soon pass.

Prolonged pressure on the acupoints is not advisable, as the nerves carrying therapeutic impulses can become over accustomed to the stimulus. Instead, each acupoint should be treated by applying a deep pressure, then releasing it. Sometimes it is more effective to position the thumb or fingertip at an angle to the point and then apply pressure. Carry out this 'pumping action' 60 times – for the duration of about a minute. The five homeostatic points (see below) should be activated twice a day, morning and evening, to maximize their preventative and curative potential. If you can get into the habit of doing it first thing in the morning and last thing at night, it will become an automatic part of your daily routine. Treatment using the other points can be administered as the need arises.

Cautions

Acupressure is a very safe form of treatment, entirely free of side effects. Even if you end up stimulating the wrong point, it will not do you any harm. However, it is important to follow certain guidelines.

- **Do not apply pressure to skin that is bruised, broken or inflamed, to open wounds or to varicose veins.**

- **The following points should not be stimulated during pregnancy: Large Intestine 4, Spleen 6, Urinary Bladder 60.**

- **Avoid acupressure treatment when under the influence of drink or recreational drugs.**

Homeostatic Points

These five points are designed to assist the process of homeostasis in our bodies. This is necessary to maintain a stable environment and to regulate the body's most important functions – blood pressure, body temperature and blood sugar levels. These are prone to be disturbed by a variety of mental and physical factors, including stress, anxiety and lack of sleep. Regular stimulation of these points will bolster your immune system, reduce allergic sensibility and keep you going through the most difficult times. Don't wait until you're run down – make it a way of life.

1. Large intestine 11 (LI 11)

Location: at the outer end of the skin crease, when the elbow is bent. Support the elbow in the fingers and palm of the opposite hand and apply deep pressure with the thumb.

Benefits: gently cleanses the digestive system and prevents and relieves constipation. Enhances the body's ability to assimilate nutrients from blood, kick-starts the metabolism and improves body shape. Tones the skin and enhances the complexion. Improves the mobility of arms and elbows. In conjunction with other points, encourages optimum functioning of all bodily systems.

2. Stomach 36 (St 36)

Location: with the knee bent at a right angle, measure four finger widths down from the lowest point of the knee. The point is at this level, one finger width towards the outside of the leg. Apply pressure with your index or middle finger.

Benefits: improves circulation throughout the body and acts as a tonic for the digestive system. By aiding digestion, it increases vitality and stamina and enhances general skin tone. Soothes tired, aching legs and feet and relieves knee joint pain.

3. Spleen 6 (Sp 6)

Location: four finger widths above the tip of the prominent bone on the inside of the ankle, just behind the shinbones. Measure with one hand and apply pressure with the middle or index finger of the other. This is where the spleen, liver and kidney meridians meet and is a very powerful acupressure point.
note: Avoid during pregnancy.

Benefits: boosts circulation and encourages elimination of excess fluids in the lower body. Raises general energy levels and enhances sexual vitality. Improves digestion and relieves abdominal bloating. Having a balancing effect on hormonal activity, it is a useful treatment for menstrual problems and premenstrual tension (PMT). Increases mobility and relieves pain in legs and feet.

4. Liver 3 (liv 3)
Location: on the upper surface of the foot, about two thumb widths below the web between the big toe and the second toe. Place your fingers under your feet and use your thumb to apply pressure in the hollow between the bones.

Benefits: improves liver function and boosts the immune system. Relieves the effect of stress and toxins in the body and regulates blood pressure. Reduces irritability sometimes referred to as 'liverishness' and combats depression. Improves circulation in legs, relieves cramp and aching muscles and helps prevent varicose veins.

5. Governing vessel 14 (GV 14)
Location: when the head is bent forward, two vertebrae stand out prominently where the top of the spine meets the base of the neck. The point is located in between the two vertebrae. Reach over your shoulder with one hand and apply firm pressure with the tip of your first or second finger, with your neck in an upright position.

Benefits: a good preventative cure-all. Highly effective in preventing illness, this point will also reinforce the other homeostatic points.

Sedative Points

These are the points that soothe the nerves and calm the mind. They are of immense value in times of stress or on any occasion when you feel anxious or agitated as they can help to minimize the internal symptoms by stimulating the discharge of tranquillizing hormones.

1. Governing vessel 20 (GV 20)

Location: in the middle of the top of the head, halfway between the ears. Position thumbs on the tips of the ears to get your bearings, then apply pressure using your middle finger.

Benefits: this is the most powerful sedative point in the body. Balances emotions and sharpens mental faculties, as well as improving the memory and powers of concentration. Very effective in regulating blood pressure and raising general energy levels.

2. Heart 7 (Ht 7)

Location: draw an imaginary straight line on the palm, starting at the web of the third (ring) finger and little finger, and finishing at the wrist. It lies at the junction of this line and the wrist crease. Support the wrist with the fingers of the opposite hand, with the palm facing upwards, and then locate the point with the thumb. Use your thumb to apply pressure with a pumping action for approximately 60 seconds.

Benefits: calms the nervous systems and relieves mental tension, anxiety and sleeplessness. A very valuable point if you are trying to give up smoking, as it strengthens and lungs and stimulates the brain to produce a chemical that makes nicotine distasteful.

3. Pericardium 6 (P 6)
Location: two thumb widths above the wrist joint, in the centre of the forearm between the tendons. Support the wrist with the fingers of the opposite hand, with the palm facing upwards, and then locate the point with the thumb. Use your thumb to apply pressure with a pumping action for approximately 60 seconds.

Benefits: calms the mind and sedates the upper digestive tract. Useful for treating nausea, vomiting (including morning sickness) and heartburn. Eases breathing difficulties triggered by anxiety and helps relieve insomnia.

4. Large Intestine 4 (LI 4)
Location: at the peak of the small mound of muscle created by pressing the thumb and first finger together. Apply firm pressure with your thumb with your fingers supporting your hand from beneath.
note: Avoid during pregnancy.

Benefits: sometimes referred to as the 'aspirin point', this general analgesic point is very effective in treating problems affecting the front of the head, the face (including all the sense organs) and the neck. Regulates the function of the lower intestine and promotes elimination. Calms the mind, relaxes the upper body and relieves tension in the neck, shoulders, arms, hands and fingers. Enhances mental function.

MASSAGE FOR FACIAL TENSION

Facial tension is something that affects us all, even though we may not be aware of it. It can manifest as a tired, lifeless complexion or wooden, expressionless features as if the muscles of your face have become frozen.

1. Tap over your face and head using the balls of your fingers – cover your cheeks, across your forehead, around your mouth and over your scalp. Work on acupressure points Large Intestine 4 and Taiyang (see page 43), which are also very effective in dissolving facial tension.

2. Continue tapping for one to two minutes to gently release the locked muscles.

Boosting Points

1. Lung 9 (Lu 9)
Location: in the shallow depression on the wrist crease at the base of the thumb on palm side. Apply pressure with your thumbs, using a pumping action for approximately 60 seconds.

Benefits: boosts respiratory system and oxygen levels. Strengthens the blood vessels in the body and brings back colour to dull complexions. Improves the suppleness of the wrists and the condition of the hands and nails.

2. Small Intestine 6 (SI 6)
Location: draw an imaginary line on the back of your hand, starting from the web between your middle and ring finger. The point is found at the junction of the line and wrist. Apply pressure with your thumb using a pumping action for approximately 60 seconds.

Benefits: relieves pain and stiffness in the neck, which helps to improve the posture. Improves the suppleness of the wrists and the condition of the hands and nails.

3. Pericardium 7 (P 7)
Location: at the centre of the inner wrist crease, between the tendons. Apply pressure with your thumb using a pumping action for about 60 seconds.

Benefits: promotes efficient circulation, which improves overall skin tone. Increases overall vitality and energy.

4. Urinary Bladder 60 (UB 60)
Location: in the hollow between the ankle bone and the Achilles tendon, on the outer side of the foot. Wrap the index finger around the ankle and apply pressure with thumb.
note: Avoid during pregnancy.

Benefits: improves function of urinary system and boosts immune system. Increases mobility and relieves aches, pains and swelling in the legs, ankles, heels and feet.

5. Gall bladder 20 (GB 20)
Location: at the back of the neck, just above the hairline, in the depression between the bottom of the skull and the neck muscles. Rest your fingers on the back of your head and apply pressure with your thumbs.

6. Taiyang
Location: one thumb width beyond the eyebrow, in a dip in the skin halfway between the outer edge of the eyebrow and the corner of the eye. Apply circular pressure using your index finger for about a minute.

Benefits: relaxes tense facial muscles and revitalizes expression and complexion.

7. Extra Point 6

Location: two finger widths above, below and to the left and right of Governing Vessel 20 (see page 34). Apply pressure with the first and second finger of each hand using a pumping action for about 60 seconds.

Benefits: relieves anxiety and insomnia and balances the mind and emotions.

Points for Enhancing Sexuality

1. Conception vessel 4
Location: measure four finger widths below the navel, and with the middle finger of the other hand apply pressure gently.

Benefits: increases sexual potency and vitality, and tones the gynaecological organs in women.

2. Conception vessel
Location: two finger widths below the navel. Use gentle rotating movements with the fingertip.

Benefits: increases energy levels and sexual vitality.

3. Urinary bladder 23
Location: on the lower back, two finger widths on either side of the spine, approximately level with the waist. Push your thumbs into the points.

Benefits: strengthens the kidneys, which are traditionally related to sexual vitality.

4. Kidney 3

Location: on the inside of the ankle in the depression just above the ankle bone. Apply pressure with your thumb, pushing slightly downwards towards the heel.

Benefits: helps increase interest in sex, if this has been lacking.

Quick-fix Acupoints

Face Revitalizer: Taiyang

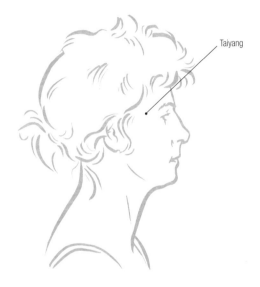

Taiyang

To relax your facial muscles and revitalize your expression:
Using your index finger, apply circular pressure to your Taiyang spot on your temples for one minute.

This is one thumb width beyond the eyebrow, in a dip in the skin halfway between the outer edge of the eyebrow and the corner of the eye.

Immunity Booster: Urinary Bladder 60

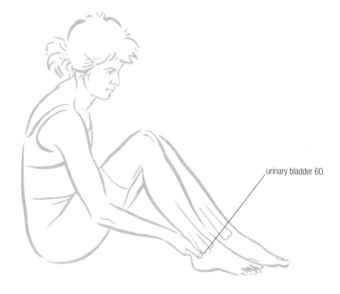

urinary bladder 60

To boost the immune system and urinary system and relieve swollen legs:

Wrap the index finger around the foot, apply pressure with the thumb to Urinary Bladder 60 on the outer side of the foot. This is located in the hollow between the ankle bone and the Achilles tendon.

note: Avoid during pregnancy.

Stress-buster: Heart 7

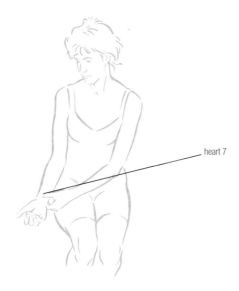

heart 7

To calm the nerves and reduce insomnia:
Support the wrist with the fingers of the opposite hand, with the palm facing upwards, then locate the point with your thumb. Use your thumb to apply pressure in a pumping action for one minute.

To find this point, draw an imaginary line on the palm, from the web between the third and little fingers to the wrist. Heart 7 is at the junction of this line and the wrist crease.

Wellbeing Cure-all: Governing Vessel 14

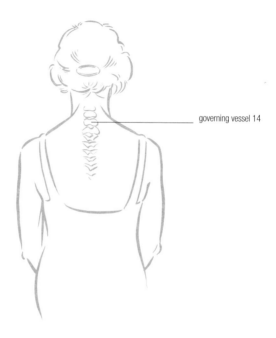

governing vessel 14

To find this point, bend your head forwards at the neck. Two vertebrae will stand out prominently where the top of the spine meets the base of your neck. The point is in the centre of these two bones. Reach over your shoulder with one hand and apply firm pressure with the tip of your first and second finger, keeping your neck upright.

Ayurvedic Massage

Ayurveda is a traditional Indian holistic therapy. It can use a combination of massage, oil therapy, yoga, herbal medicines and meditation. It functions on two levels – as a system of illness prevention, and also as a medical science – the literal translation of Ayurveda is 'the science of life'. As with many complementary health techniques, and as with medical science, it involves many years of study.

The philosophies that underpin Ayurveda were cemented by sages, or Rishis, of India more than 3000 years ago. They felt it necessary to remove themselves from the stress of daily living in order to meditate upon the diseases that afflict all creatures and prevent enlightenment. A committed group of them gathered together in the foothills of the Himalayas and wrote down the insights that came to them. Some insights were said to be divinely inspired, others from their collective contemplation. These combined instructions – found in the best-known Ayurvedic text, the Charaka Samhita – form the basis of modern Ayurveda.

Ayurveda's focus on cleansing and purification (Panchakarma) and rejuvenation (Rasayana) is a great counterbalance to our stressed out, polluted urban lives. In the West, we are caught up with making money, calorie-counting, staying slim and looking young. We relieve the stress all this creates by drinking alcohol, smoking and taking drugs, and then try to salvage our ravaged bodies with quick trips to the health farm, expensive creams and facelifts, and a great deal of angst and frustration.

But Ayurveda views life in a more honest way. It focuses on listening to your mind and body and understanding what it wants, and helps to rebalance using natural remedies and simple exercises. The science makes a clear connection between emotional distress and physical deterioration. This holistic view suggests that illness affects both mind and body, and both should be treated together. If you have a headache or back pain it is only natural that it will affect your mental wellbeing. Equally, your mood also feeds your state of health – if you are depressed you are more prone to suffer physical complaints, because you may find it harder to care for yourself or eat as sensibly as you should. Conversely, if you are happy and buoyant you are less likely to fall ill.

What's your Ayurvedic Type?

Ayurvedic practitioners believe that an imbalance in one area of health can result in a number of different problems depending on the background of the afflicted individual. This can be seen by classifying everyone according to three fundamental types.

At the heart of Ayurveda is the concept that there are three universal governing forces at work inside us all. These are called the doshas and they are described as Fire, Air and Earth. They are in a state of continual flux at work inside all of us, but there is a tendency for one or two to dominate in each person. You are created with an inborn doshic disposition that affects not only your physical characteristics – body shape, skin type, colouring and metabolism – but also your emotional and mental temperament. Your individual type (known as your prakriti) can in turn give clues about the types of illnesses you are most likely to suffer from, and help you begin to take steps to avoid them. Ayurveda sees illness as a result of disturbances in your doshic type.

Using Massage Oils in Ayurveda

In Ayurvedic oil treatment, oils are specially selected to balance your doshic type. These are massaged into the skin (see cards 10–20 and 27–30), during which any blockages in the marma points on the body are released. Marmas are akin to acupuncture points in Chinese medicine, and Ayurveda identifies 107 marma points in an energy matrix throughout the body, through which the prana – or life force – flows.

To select Ayurvedic oils for your particular dosha, first read below to see which profile most describes you and your lifestyle. Remember that pure single-type people are uncommon; most of us will have a dominant and secondary dosha. For example, Nicole Kidman's doshic type is Air-Fire, with Air being her dominant dosha and Fire, her secondary dosha. So you will need to read the massage oils and touch recommendations for both of your doshas.

Air (vata) types

Air types are natural whirlwinds, energetic and unpredictable. You are artistic, oversensitive at times and can be prone to burnout. At your best, you can be creative and visionary, but when you overload yourself you experience digestive problems, you get scatty, prone to sensitive, dry skin, sleepless nights and you become less effective. You need to avoid crash-and-burn by making more time to relax, and try to adopt a few elements of routine into your life – Tai Chi, walking, dancing, yoga. Air types include Gwyneth Paltrow, Leonardo di Caprio and Julia Roberts.

Fire (pitta) types

You are one of life's alchemists, blazing a trail, making a difference. You are as fiery and passionate as your type name suggests – dynamic and inspirational. When your life is in balance you have the attractive, commanding presence of a natural leader, radiating perception, love taking control and encouraging others to have a good time. But if you overdo it, you can become critical, brittle, overly competitive and your skin can flare up as a visual indication of your internal combustion. Non-competitive sports such as swimming and cycling will give you the physical expression you require. Learn the art of compromise and make time to relax. Fire types include Jennifer Aniston, Marco Pierre White and Cindy Crawford.

Earth (kapha) types

At your best you are as grounded and dependable as your type suggests – solid, patient and intensely loyal. You are drawn towards people, who in turn confide in you, and you're wonderful in a crisis. When you're out of balance, that laid back charm can turn into sluggishness and your skin can become excessively oily. You can vegetate, seeking solace in yet more chocolate and feeling stagnant internally. If you feel this happening you need to act fast: eat fresh fruit and vegetables. Running, tennis and aerobics will get your metabolism moving again. Earth types include Oprah Winfrey, Kate Winslet and Dawn French.

What's the Right Oil for your Type?

Ayurvedic massage is particularly effective because, rather than using a generic oil for everyone, there are massage oils geared to perfection for each type, which have been formulated and handed down over the millennia. The right massage oil for your type will nourish your skin, reduce fatigue and stress, improve metabolism and slow the effects of ageing, while adding lustre to the skin and hair. It also helps the body by detoxification and promotes a sense of tranquillity and wellbeing.

Air types should use calming oils: sesame, olive, almond, wheatgerm and castor oils.

Fire types should use cooling oils: sunflower, almond, coconut and sandalwood oils.

Earth types should use invigorating oils: mustard, corn or canola oils.

Warming the oil before you begin

Oils for Ayurvedic massage should be warmed before use. To do this, measure half a cup of your chosen oil and heat in a microwave. The oil should be warm and comfortable to the touch. It should never boil – apart from the damage this would do to your skin, boiling the oil changes its properties and makes it less effective. Therefore, if you boil the oil accidentally, discard it rather than leaving it to cool before application. If you don't have a microwave, let the oil warm gently in a heatproof dish over a pan of simmering water.

Aromatherapy in Ayruveda

Essential oils used in aromatherapy are highly volatile aromatic oils, produced by plants in order to attract insects and fight off disease. When our brain detects the presence of these oils we experience a powerful response that subconsciously influences our memory, emotions and libido.

Using aromatherapy oils in Ayurvedic massage follows the 'opposites attract' theory – you calm an inflamed Fire type with cooling oils; you reinvigorate a sluggish Earth type with a stimulating oil; you soothe stress for Air types with a calming balm.

Air types: Ylang ylang, patchouli, geranium, lavender, cedar wood and myrrh.

Earth types: Frankincense, sage, rosemary, camphor, basil and eucalyptus.

Fire types: Saffron, jasmine, rose, sandalwood, gardenia and lotus.

For face oil, add 25 drops of essential oil to 25ml of base oil (this can be ghee, vegetable oil or one of the massage oils listed above). Dab a few drops of face oil on your cupped hand, add a sprinkle of water and apply to moist skin.

For body oil, add 10 drops of essential oil to 25ml of base oil, and again apply to moist skin.

Ayurvedic Massage Techniques

Using the massage cards, try these three sequences that work as great Ayurvedic oil treatments: the friction massage (Cards 26–28), the rejuvenating face massage (Cards 10–15) and the scalp massage (Cards 16–20). You can use the massage oil or aromatherapy massage oil recommended for your type for these sequences.

For the friction massage (see Cards 26–28) you can also choose a particular type of touch to benefit your doshic type.

Dry skin – Air types: Use a 'sattvic' touch, which is light, calm and slow. Too much pressure aggravates Air types and will lead to feelings of unsettled agitation.

Sensitive skin – Fire types: Use a 'rajasic' touch, moderate pressure and speed but not too much so fiery types are not aggravated.

Oily skin – Earth types: Use a 'tamasic' touch. This is deep and vigorous and ensures stimulation for slower Earth natures.

For the scalp massage, try this delicious potion for hair lustre oil, which makes your hair soft and gleaming. Generations of Indian mothers have passed this on to their daughters.

- **Pour two teaspoons of natural coconut oil into a saucepan.**

- **Heat gently and add a splash of rosewater or a handful of real rose petals.**

- **Add a little masala spice powder, cover with a lid and simmer for three minutes. When cool, coat your hair in this beautifully fragrant concoction or pour onto your scalp in sections as described in the scalp massage (Cards 16–20). Leave for one hour, then shampoo and wash in the usual way. Your hair will have a wonderful lustre and scent.**

Heart and Soul: Massage and the Chakras

Chakras are the symbolic representations of the body's endocrine glands, or hormonal centres, and are sometimes known as 'energy wheels'. They work together, striving for balance in mind and body. During massage, the chakra points are stimulated and rebalanced, which gives a great healing boost to body and mind together.

There are seven principal chakra points on the body, and all have particular emotional and spiritual associations. They are located at the crown of the head, the third eye between the eyebrows, the throat, heart, solar plexus, navel and root, at the genitals.

Everyone can experience the feeling of the chakras without being aware of their origin. When you feel the sensation of butterflies in your stomach before a significant event, or become aware of a knot in your throat when you feel emotional but can't express yourself, or feel that delicious melting sexual arousal in your lower body, you are literally sensing the effect of your chakras. When you are waiting for the person you love at an airport and finally see them emerge, the physical feeling of warmth in your chest is your heart chakra reflecting the love that resides within you.

Each chakra is known by a different colour – the colour that symbolizes its function. Becoming aware of your chakras and concentrating on each one in turn for a few minutes will help give you a reading about the state of your emotional and physical health.

The red chakra

This is the sexual centre. It is located in the genitals and is associated with life and survival. When energy flows through it, you feel infused with passionate direction, aliveness, alertness and sexual desire. When the energy is blocked you can feel guilt about sex, emotionally needy and directionless.

The orange chakra

This is the lower body chakra, located just below the navel, and is the body's centre of balance and movement. Strength, vitality and physical grace flow through this chakra. But if the energy becomes blocked here, you can feel hypercritical, stiff, tense and aggressive.

The yellow chakra

This is the solar plexus chakra, located in the hollow just below the rib cage. This is the centre of our self-esteem. Charisma, radiance, cheerfulness, self-confidence and a sense of possibility and new horizons are experiences that flow from here. When blocked, we feel nervous, timid and unconfident.

The green chakra

This is the heart chakra, located in the centre of the chest. When energy flows here we really fly, we feel love, joy, playfulness and laughter coupled with trust, compassion and empathy. But close this chakra up and we are left with great negativity, doubt, cynicism and bitterness.

The violet chakra

This is located in the throat, and is our centre of self-determination and personal authenticity. We can give voice to our needs and desire when energy flows through here, we stand up for what we believe in, we demonstrate integrity in our feelings – even if that involves appearing anti-social or obstinate. Take away the energy from this centre and we are left directionless, we become listless, worthless and constantly put our partner's needs above our own. We feel that life is only skin deep and cannot touch us more deeply.

The blue chakra

This is located on the forehead, between and behind the eyebrows. This is the third eye, that part of ourselves that makes us feel free, creative, imaginative and intuitive – having insight without needing to use logic and reason. Block this centre and life seems dull and listless, devoid of meaning or higher purpose or personal fulfilment.

The white chakra

This is also known as the crown chakra, and is located on top of the head. This is the most magical of all the chakras. When the energy flows here we feel sensations of complete fulfilment and pure joy – it creates a delicious connection to everyone and everything in which we are at our best, most spontaneous and evolved selves. We feel invincible, capable of achieving whatever goals we set ourselves. But close this centre and you are exiled to an insubstantial fantasy world grasping at the beauty that lies beyond the screen, unable to feel spiritually authentic or truly connected to yourself or your partner.

4 ADDITIONAL MASSAGES

Ear massage for all-over vitality and radiance

The relationship between the ear and internal organs was first recorded more than 2000 years ago in Chinese medical texts. Massaging your ear has enormous health benefits. Giving yourself an auricular massage improves the quality of the whole body. First, remove earrings. Let your ear guide you to the treatment you require. Press quite hard, and where you have a weakness you will find that your ear hurts at the corresponding point. Do not avoid the area: let the tenderness be your guide to what area of your body needs attention – this applies to all areas treated with acupressure. For an effective holistic treatment of the entire body, follow these simple massage instructions.

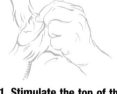

1. Stimulate the top of the ear. This helps with weakness of the diaphragm. Massaging the groove under the top of the ear is good for lowering blood pressure.

2. Work your way around the ear, making a sequence of deep pinches, and rolling the cartilage between your thumb and forefinger.

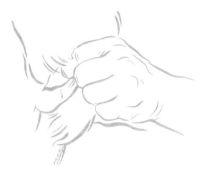

3. Pull on the flange of the ear to stimulate the meridian point that corresponds to the liver. Manipulate it using the fingerball method – see Card 1.

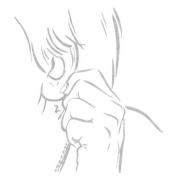

4. Press on the node in front of the ear to stimulate the lungs and heart, helping to oxygenate the body and improve circulation.

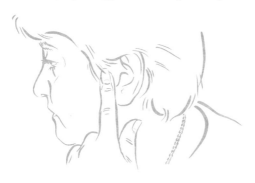

5. With firm pressure, press in the middle of the ear, against the cartilage. This stimulates the adrenal gland, which has a strong influence over the body's hormonal system.

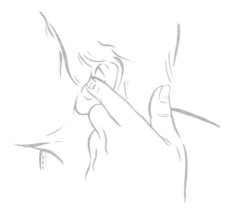

6. Stretch the ear forward to stimulate the back of the ear.

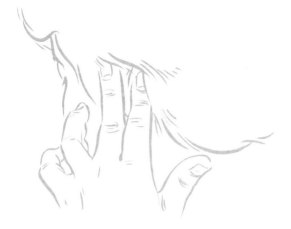

Circulation-boosting foot massage

This massage improves your circulation, which encourages all your systems to work more effectively. It improves digestion, encourages the elimination of water retention and abdominal bloating, while raising energy levels and enhancing sexual vitality. It also has a balancing effect on hormonal activity, and is useful for treating PMT. Direct stimulation of the feet also helps relieve aches, pains and swelling in the legs, ankles, heels and feet.

Work on each foot for around five minutes. Begin on the weakest foot, the one that feels more tender to the touch.

1. Press on the three points shown using the third (ring) finger, middle finger and index finger. Move your fingers upwards, maintaining a deep pressure to encourage improved circulation.

2. The area surrounding the inner ankle bone is very important. Apply deep fingerball pressure to stimulate the spleen and kidney meridians, which are very important points in Chinese medicine. Applying acupressure here leads to detoxification, helps to remove waste products, gives hormonal balance and allows the tissues to work better. Working on the inside of the ankle can also ease dryness of the vagina and help decrease high blood pressure.

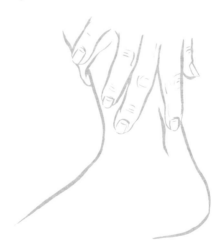

3. If the inside of the leg is too sensitive, keep working, but decrease the pressure as you move your fingers up the leg to a point four finger widths above the tip of the ankle bone. Be careful to avoid bruising yourself. Even working gently on the thinner skin on this very powerful acupoint is beneficial, as it is the meeting point of the spleen, liver and kidney meridians. It tones and strengthens the gynaecological organs and helps to keep them in position.

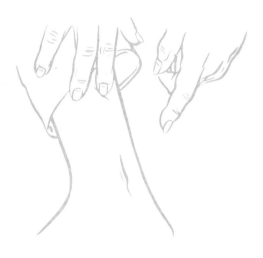

4. The base of the fleshy part of the underside of your foot is a good acupressure pump and is found in the depression just below the ball of the foot. Pressing deeply for up to a minute, and letting go several times helps to invigorate the circulation, promotes vitality, helps to balance blood pressure and is a good treatment for older people as it increases blood flow to all areas.

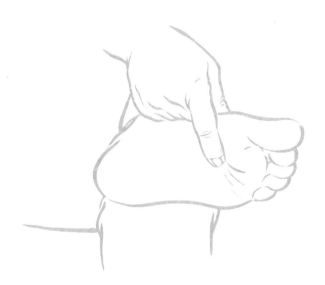

5. This is splint 6; in Chinese medicine it is recognized as the strongest point for controlling the hormones. To find it, mark out your four fingers from the ankle bone as a guide. Press your thumb into the point using deep pressure before letting go. Repeat this several times. Working on the outside of the ankle can also benefit the ovaries.

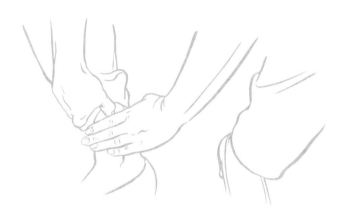

6. The area surrounding the bone is very important, and can help to reduce high blood pressure. Use concentrated deep fingerball pressure (see Card 1).

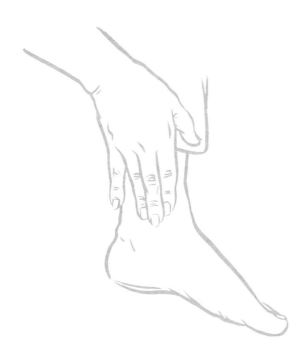

7. These points on the foot shown in the illustration below are very important for blood pressure. Press with quite a deep pressure, and then drag your finger away to give a boost to your circulation. Working on the front of the foot also improves liver function and boosts the immune system. Pull your fingers firmly along the top of the foot to intercept the nerve junction. Repeat this process to relieve the effects of stress and toxins in the body, and to regulate blood pressure.

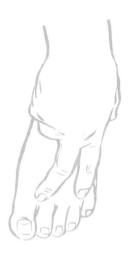
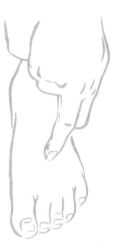

Stress-busting hand massage

Easy to perform at any time of the day, even when travelling or at work, this massage calms the nervous system and treats the hormonal system, producing a feeling of calm. Further benefits include easing sleeplessness and digestive problems, harmonizing the breath, and improving hand and nail condition.

1. The fleshy part of the hand is very important in acupressure. Massage here benefits the whole body, particularly the skin and complexion. The area is also a good general tonic acupoint, which promotes circulation, the flow of energy and good digestion. Think of this area as a pump, which, when stimulated, helps activate circulation.

Using the thumb of the other hand, press firmly down on the fleshy pad between forefinger and thumb, moving from the base of the thumb towards the wrist.

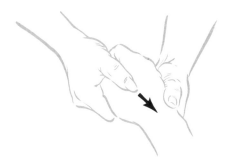

2. Using a firm rocking pressure, move your thumb up inside the wrist.

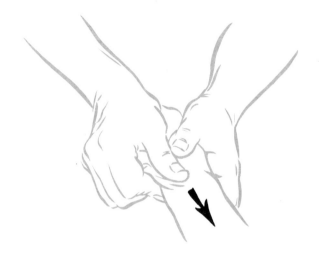

3. Apply pressure to the point two finger widths from the wrist crease in the depression behind the bone, and angle the pressure slightly down towards the wrist and thumb. Apply sustained pressure and fingerballs for a minute; this action will strengthen the respiratory system.

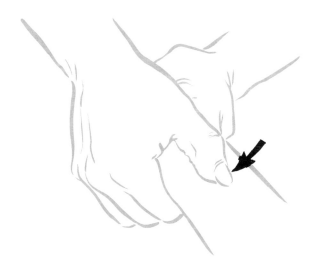

4. Apply fingerballs to the middle of the palm between the bones leading to the index and middle fingers; then apply pressure angled slightly towards the middle fingers to calm the mind and reduce feelings of stress and irritability.

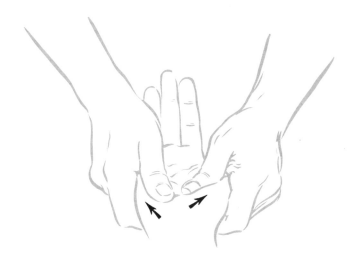

5. In the middle of the wrist crease, apply pressure angling your touch towards the palm of the hand. Press in between the blood vessels and tendons – not directly on them – to promote circulation. This action also helps relieve any faintness caused by anxiety.

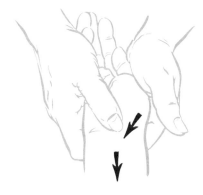

6. Move the thumb three finger widths from the wrist crease. Apply pressure with the balls of your fingers to calm the mind and relieve anxiety.

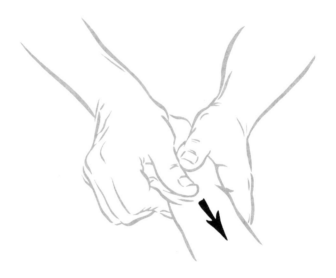

7. Apply pressure to the three points along the wrist line – left, centre and right – to improve circulation, ease breathing, strengthen heart function, calm the mind and help you sleep.

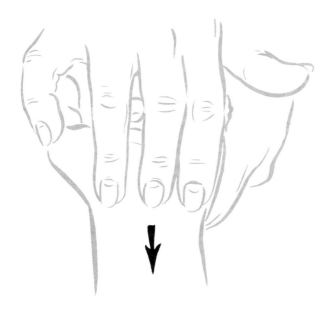

8. Move your fingers three finger widths further up the arm towards the elbow. Apply gentle pressure angled slightly downwards for 30 to 60 seconds. This stimulates and regulates the heart, and promotes good circulation of blood and energy.

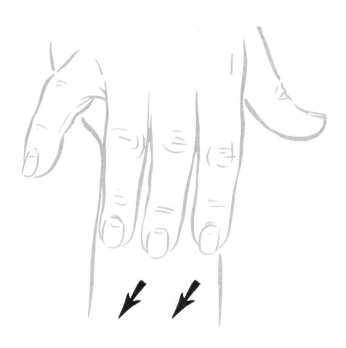

Anti-cellulite massage

Cellulite is the hard, lumpy, dimpled 'orange peel' effect that appears on upper arms, bottoms and thighs. It's visual evidence that there is waste from the metabolic process left in the body. It doesn't happen overnight – it is actually a slow process that develops over many years. There are three processes that, when used together over a period of time, can help reduce cellulite: a detoxifying diet, regular body polishing to stimulate the circulation and lymphatic drainage massage upon the bulges.

This intensive lymphatic drainage massage is a pain-free, but vigorous, pummelling massage, focused specifically upon areas of cellulite, that loosens the build-up of toxins. It also activates the lymph nodes, helping to transport toxins away from the affected area.

1. Body polishing helps loosen the fat, without damaging the blood vessels, before you begin the intensive massage. Moisten your hands with water. Place your palms flat against your skin and let them glide over every contour of your body. First, polish up the back of the leg using long strokes. At the thigh, stroke repeatedly to shift the stubborn areas of accumulated toxins within the cellulite. You can also palm the buttocks (see Card 2) in a circular direction to keep pimples at bay, which are caused by follicles becoming irritated from a lot of sitting down. Then move onto the front of your thighs, followed by arms, torso and neck.

2. Take a bath and add a few drops of aromatherapy oil to the water. Choose from lemon, frankincense, juniper, black pepper and sandalwood – these oils have a great detoxifying effect on the body. While you are still in the bath, pummel and knead the cellulite-heavy areas. When you've finished, get out of the bath and massage a diluted droplet of your chosen oil into your thighs and buttocks. The oils will take about 10 minutes to be absorbed completely.

3. Touch the lymph nodes under the armpits, around the groin and behind the knees to boost the functioning of your lymphatic system. Apply gentle pressure until any tenderness there ceases. Follow this routine every day. After three or four weeks, use the oils every other day. When you can see a noticeable change or improvement in your cellulite, you can cut down to once or twice a week. You do, however, need to complement this routine with a change in your eating habits in order to see a change to your cellulite.

Sensuality massage

This is a very intimate and therapeutic 10-minute massage that has the power to change the energy between you and your partner. It can be used as part of foreplay, or simply to create a stronger emotional connection between you. Here the woman takes the active role, but once you have shown your partner this massage, encourage him to massage you first. After making love, when he is falling asleep, you can then massage him – as a woman, you will be left with a lot more energy!

1. Take a bath together, or bathe independently if you prefer. While your partner is still in the water, begin massaging the top of his spine at the base of his neck, using the fingerball method (see Card 1).

2. Dry each other and sit naked on the bed. Apply some body lotion or an aromatherapy oil blend to his back (see page 56). Continue to work up and down his spine, varying the pressure between feathering (see Card 2), pinching (see Card 3) and fingerballing. Gradually he will want to relax and lie down.

3. Encourage him to lie on his stomach. Straddle his buttocks so your genitals touch his bottom, reminding him of the warmth and pleasure of your body. Place your hands upon the fleshy part of his buttocks. This is an important gall bladder pressure point. Invigorate the area by pressing firmly upon the buttocks and

pushing up towards his spine. Repeat this many times, using a deep pressure. This acts like a blood pump, and will boost the circulation and increase sexual vitality.

4. Using the balls of your fingers, place each hand two inches either side of the vertebrae. Use your knuckles to penetrate into the connective tissue and roll them around, using quite a lot of pressure, which is very soothing.

5. Alternate this with sensuous palming (see Card 2), stroking his body before working more deeply upon the areas you have prepared. Use the palms of your hands to gently stroke your partner, particularly on the inside of his thighs and the soles of his feet.

6. To close the massage, place the flat of your palm at the top of his spine and pass it very lightly down the full length. Do this 10 times to soothe your partner, who may now be feeling very sensual.

Face massage for intimacy

This gentle massage takes only 15 minutes to perform and has added benefits if you choose to work through it with your partner. If you feel in a rut sexually, or always feel under pressure to have full sex, this massage can make a very energizing change. The massage-performing partner sits with their back to a sofa, wall or headboard, with a large cushion placed in their lap. The passive partner lies back, fully clothed, with their head resting in the centre of the cushion. Take a small amount of oil, lotion or an aphrodisiac aromatherapy blend such as jojoba and bergamot, and caress your lover's face, spreading oil out smoothly. Keeping your touch light, sensuous, and slow, move your fingers over their forehead, down their cheeks, around the nose and across the under-eye area to finish past the ears. Continue for 15 minutes, then change places. Remember that, in this tender voyage of romantic discovery, neither of you need remove your clothes or even speak to feel these sensual benefits.

Good Nutrition

Practising massage and acupressure techniques puts you uniquely in tune with your body, working from the outside in. It is natural, too, to want to nurture your body from the inside out. Many of us, however, stockpile the kitchen with fabulous organic produce for a health-fest without considering the need for dietary balance – which is, after all, what our bodies strive for at every level. The old adage of a 'healthy, balanced diet' means just that – balancing your intake of proteins, carbohydrates, fruits and vegetables and fats to allow you to enjoy optimum health.

Although your appetite may tell you otherwise, you need a larger proportion of some types of food than others. (There is also a great deal of evidence to suggest that a meat-free diet, or one that includes little meat, leaves more room for foods that help the body run more smoothly rather than adding to its burden.) Below is a sample eating plan to take you through the day, with recommended servings for each food type.

DAILY FOOD PLAN

bread, rice, pasta, cereal, potatoes
6 servings. For example: 2 slices bread, 3 heaped tablespoons of cooked rice or pasta, 90g (3½ oz) cooked potato.

fruit and vegetables
5 servings. For example: small glass freshly squeezed fruit or vegetable juice, small mixed salad, 2 tablespoons of steamed vegetables.

fish, poultry, meat, eggs, nuts, seeds, pulses
2 servings. For example: 75g (3 oz) oily fish, 300g (12 oz) cooked pulses.

milk, cheese, yoghurt
2 servings. For example: 200ml (⅓ pint) milk, small pot of yoghurt.

water
8–10 glasses.

fats
1 tablespoon of 'good' fats and oils, such as olive or sesame oils, rather than saturated fats (see page 92).

Essential Nutrients

Carbohydrates

Carbohydrates supply the energy needed for day-to-day running of the body. Ideally, carbohydrates should make up half of your diet. Slow-burning, complex carbohydrates such as fruits, vegetables and grains, eaten regularly, help keep you on an even keel, both physically and emotionally. Choose wholegrains and unrefined cereals for maximum fibre and goodness, and eat a variety of cereals and grains.

Try:

* **Oaty mueslis and cereals or porridge for a sustaining breakfast.**

* **Brown rice and cracked wheat, cooked and left to cool, as a base for salads.**

* **Rye bread made with mixed grains.**

* **Soba noodles and buckwheat pasta.**

* **Rice cakes, oatcakes and rye crispbreads.**

* **Cornmeal for baking and to make polenta – a perfect accompaniment for grilled foods.**

Fruit and vegetables

Fruit and vegetables are a vital source of vitamins, minerals, fibre and water. These foods nourish and cleanse the body and protect it from disease. Vitamin C strengthens collagen, capillaries and your immune system. Vitamin C, beta-carotene and vitamin E neutralize the effect of free radicals – the body's internal cell saboteurs. Beta-carotene is the yellow–orange pigment found in foods such as carrots, mangoes and apricots; avocado and kiwi fruit are a good source of vitamin E.

All fruits and vegetables contain potassium, which helps regulate fluid balance in cells and tissues, combating fluid retention and bloating.

Try:

- **Eating raw fruits and vegetables to get the maximum nutritional benefit and for their dynamic internal cleansing action.**

- **Including a salad with nearly every meal.**

- **Plenty of iron-rich spinach, watercress and parsley to keep up your haemoglobin level, particularly just before a period and during pregnancy.**

- Snacking on sweet fruits for some instant vitality. Bananas are particularly good energy-boosters.

- Feeding your nails, teeth and bones by eating dark-green vegetables, such as cabbage and broccoli – they're a great source of calcium.

Protein

Protein is vital to a good diet, but the body needs only a modest amount – around 55g ($2^{1}/_{4}$ oz) per day. Excessive consumption overloads the liver and kidneys – the vital organs of detoxification – and can result in the loss of certain minerals, especially calcium, and an increased risk of osteoporosis. Good sources of protein include lean cuts of meat, poultry, fish, milk, eggs, cheese, dried peas, beans, chick peas, lentils, nuts (unsalted), sesame, sunflower and pumpkin seeds, cereals (especially wheatgerm) and potatoes.

Try:

- **Poultry and game, which have less fat than other meats.**

- **Eating at least two portions of fish each week. Oily fish and shellfish also help keep skin moist and strengthen hair and nails.**

- **Snacking on pumpkin, sesame and sunflower seeds, which are packed with protein, fibre and skin-replenishing nutrients.**

- **Combining nuts and seeds, pulses and wholegrains in nutritious snacks for a low-fat, high-fibre protein boost: peanut butter or beans on wholegrain toast, or pitta bread with hummus.**

Fats

Fats are essential to health, and should represent 30 per cent of food intake. They are needed to absorb the fat-soluble vitamins A, D, E and K, and provide protective padding for delicate organs and bony areas of the body. Fats are a concentrated source of energy, and therefore calories, so we need to choose dietary fats carefully, avoiding saturated fats and choosing reduced-fat dairy products and small amounts of monounsaturated and polyunsaturated fats (EFAs). EFAs are found in avocados, olive oil, sunflower oil, seeds and oily fish.

Try:

- **Eating butter in moderation, along with margarines labelled 'unhydrogenated', as these have not been subjected to the solidifying process that causes them to behave more like saturated fats. There is a clear link between heavy consumption of saturated fats (found in butter, hard cheese and red meat) and heart disease.**

- **Using oils that are cold-pressed and unrefined – that is, nutritionally intact. If you need to fry at a high temperature use olive or sesame oils, which remain stable in a hot pan (don't, however, heat to 'smoking' point, which depletes the nutritional value of the oil). For gentle frying or sautéing, use corn or sunflower oil.**

- **Buying soft cheeses and sheep- or goat-milk cheeses.**

About Wheat and Dairy Products

Try not to allow wheat and dairy products to dominate your diet. Gluten, the gummy protein in wheat, and mucus-forming milk, cream, cheese and butter have a tendency to clog up the intestines and interfere with nutrient absorption. Tell-tale signs of congestion include a general feeling of sluggishness and an increase in the frequency of colds and other mucusy conditions. There is often expansion around the midriff, too, not accompanied by weight gain elsewhere.

Excluding wheat and diary products from your diet for three months will firm up and trim your figure, breathe new life into your skin and increase your general vitality, by improving your digestion and assimilation of food and keeping your respiratory system clear. It can take up to seven weeks to loosen the build-up in the intestines, which leaves five weeks or more for the therapeutic effects to be felt. In cases of very heavy congestion, a six-month period is recommended. Repeat every five years or so, as the need arises.

Wheat Products

Bread
Pasta
Most cakes and biscuits
Many breakfast cereals
Semolina, couscous
Bulgur (cracked wheat)
Wheatgerm and bran

Wheat Alternatives

100 per cent rye bread and crispbread
Rice (grains, cakes, noodles)
Potatoes
Oats (oatcakes, porridge, oatbran)
Corn (polenta, tortillas, cornflakes)
Buckwheat pasta and pancakes
Popcorn, poppadoms, corn chips
Cornflour, potato flour, arrowroot
 (thickeners)

Dairy Products

Milk
Butter
Some margarines
Cheese
Yoghurt

Dairy Alternatives

Goat's milk/cheese/yoghurt
Sheep's milk/cheese/yoghurt
Soya milk/yoghurt, tofu
Non-dairy margarine
Mayonnaise
Cold-pressed oils
Tahini
Hummus